GINSENG

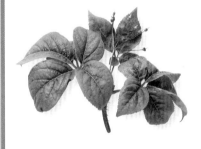

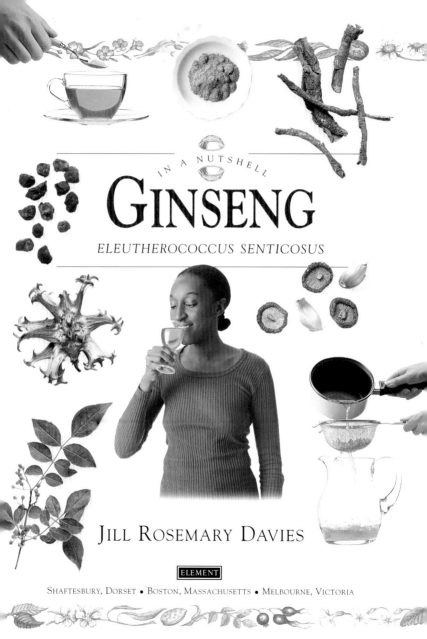

IN A NUTSHELL

GINSENG

ELEUTHEROCOCCUS SENTICOSUS

JILL ROSEMARY DAVIES

ELEMENT

SHAFTESBURY, DORSET • BOSTON, MASSACHUSETTS • MELBOURNE, VICTORIA

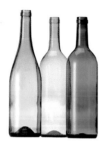

© Element Books Limited 1999

First published in Great Britain in 1999 by
ELEMENT BOOKS LIMITED
Shaftesbury, Dorset SP7 8BP

Published in the USA in 1999 by
ELEMENT BOOKS INC.
160 North Washington Street,
Boston MA 02114

Published in Australia in 1999 by
ELEMENT BOOKS LIMITED
and distributed by
Penguin Australia Ltd
487 Maroondah Highway,
Ringwood, Victoria 3134

NOTE FROM THE PUBLISHER
Any information given in this book is not
intended to be taken as a replacement for
medical advice. Any person with a condition
requiring medical attention should consult
a qualified practitioner or therapist.
For growing and harvesting, calendar
information applies only to the northern
hemisphere (US zones 5–9).

Jill Rosemary Davies has asserted her right
under the Copyright, Designs, and Patents
Act, 1988, to be identified as Author of
this work.

Designed and created for Element Books with
The Bridgewater Book Company Ltd.

ELEMENT BOOKS LIMITED
Managing Editor Miranda Spicer
Senior Commissioning Editor Caro Ness
Group Production Director Clare Armstrong
Production Manager Susan Sutterby

THE BRIDGEWATER BOOK COMPANY
Editorial Director Sophie Collins
Project Editor Lorraine Turner
Art Director Kevin Knight
Designer Jane Lanaway
DTP Designer Chris Lanaway
Photography Guy Ryecart
Illustrations Michael Courtney
Three-dimensional models Mark Jamieson
Picture research Lynda Marshall

Printed and bound in Great Britain by
Butler & Tanner, Frome

Library of Congress Cataloging in
Publication data available

British Library Cataloguing in Publication
data available

ISBN 1 86204 505 4

The publishers wish to thank the
following for the use of pictures:
A–Z Botanical Collection: pp.24b, 25.
Bridgeman Art Library: p.10, Krasnoyarskiy
Kraevoy Musey, Krasnoyarsk, Russia; 38,
Private Collection.
Image Bank: pp.6t, 9t, 11c, 15t, 20b, 21, 26,
28, 40.
Science Photo Library: pp.14t, 16, 18b,
22, 53t.
Stock Market: pp.23, 42, 45, 52t.

Contents

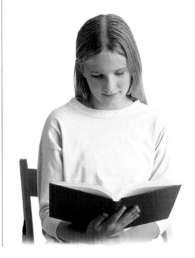

Introduction

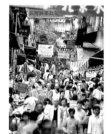

THE WORD GINSENG means "the wonder of the world." This herb is an ancient tonic from the Far East and is widely used to treat a diverse range of illnesses.

LEFT **Eastern medicine uses Ginseng for its tonic effect.**

DEFINITION

Botanical family: Araliaceae
Species: *Eleutherococcus senticosus*
In botanical terms *Eleutherococcus senticosus* is not a true Ginseng, but it acts exactly like one as a balancing and energizing tonic – and it has no known side effects.

M any varieties of Ginseng are grown in China, Korea, Russia, and the United States, but this book will concentrate on Siberian Ginseng. Highly honored in the East, Siberian Ginseng's recent revival in the West is quite understandable given its profound ability to balance and "normalize" the body – physically and mentally – and therefore help people to cope with stressful events and everyday tensions.

Siberian Ginseng is classified as an adaptogen, which means it helps the body adapt to stress. It is one of the best herbs for helping recovery from illness and for maintaining good health, mostly by stimulating and sustaining resistance to stress.

BELOW **Eleutherococcus senticosus** *is from a different plant family to other Ginsengs.*

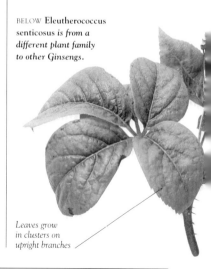

Leaves grow in clusters on upright branches

Siberian Ginseng is a tall, striking shrub that grows to 5–7ft (1½–2m) in height. Its leaves look like those of horse-chestnut trees, with three to five small, toothed leaves at the end of each stalk, which are borne on upright branches. The young shoots have long, thick, brown "prickles."

Mature stems are straight with sharp, fragile thorns that protrude downward. At first, the light grayish-brown branches are densely covered with thorns, but the thorns diminish as the years pass. The shrub can grow for up to 100 years, but even at this age it continues to produce offspring.

The flowers appear in July as magnificent umbels of clustered cream stars. In the wild, the color can vary to pale yellow, lilac, or violet. The flowers are followed in the fall by striking clusters of black berries.

Siberian Ginseng has three types of reproductive system: male, female, and bisexual, something of a botanical curiosity, which emphasizes its adaptive and fiercely procreative abilities.

Shoots have long prickles and stems have thorns

THE GINSENG FAMILY

Red Ginseng (Latin name *Panax*, Chinese name *Ren shen*) is a "warmer," more stimulating Ginseng, and is predominantly used for men. It should be used only for short periods of time, when energy is very depleted, and under the direction of a qualified herbalist or medical practitioner. While some strong, active people do take it regularly, for example athletes, there is genuine concern that it can be over-used and cause side effects such as high blood pressure.

There is also a white version of Red Ginseng, but it is less powerful. Botanically the same species, both are therapeutic for a wide variety of conditions from infertility to digestive problems and mild diabetes.

American Ginseng (*Panax quinquefolium*) is often used in similar situations as Siberian Ginseng. Although American Ginseng has more stimulating qualities, it lacks the balance that the adaptogenic Siberian Ginseng is able to bring to the body.

American Ginseng is less powerful than Red Ginseng, but it can be taken safely over a longer period of time.

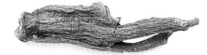

REN SHEN

Exploring Siberian Ginseng

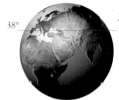

SIBERIAN GINSENG IS a hardy plant and can grow in full sun or in the shade. It is found in cool zones north of latitude 38°, most often in terrain over 2,600ft (800m) above sea level.

38°

LEFT *Siberian Ginseng grows in the northern hemisphere.*

WHERE TO FIND SIBERIAN GINSENG

Siberian Ginseng grows abundantly in the wild in parts of Russia (notably Siberia), Mongolia, Korea, China, and Japan. It thrives in mountainous, forested regions with a mixture of evergreen and deciduous trees. While the plant will quickly proliferate in any clearings where it can find full sun, it is also adept at jostling in the thickest parts of the woods, where there is little or even no sun. A tough survivor, it has the ability to adapt to many different situations in order to procreate. One of its survival mechanisms is to create an impenetrable fortification of thorns to keep out other species of plants or animals.

COMMERCIAL GROWERS

The most prolific commercial source of Siberian Ginseng is China. The herb also grows throughout Siberia and elsewhere in Asia, but here the wild root of the plant is more likely to be used. Wild roots are the best quality, so generally these remain in their country of origin rather than being exported. Small commercial quantities are also being grown in other areas, including the US and Scotland.

SOIL REQUIREMENTS

Being a woodland plant, Siberian Ginseng prefers leaf mold and humus-rich soils, where

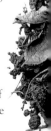

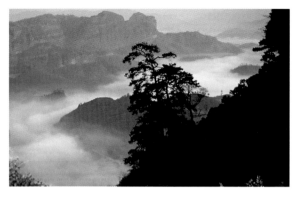

LEFT *Ginseng plants need plenty of water, so they tend to flourish in moist woodland areas.*

its webbing rhizomes can make easy networks in the soft, fertile earth. In China, commercial farms favor loamy to acidic soils, with leaf mold added if necessary. When providing the plant with a suitable soil, it is important to remember its ability to hold water, because it needs plenty of year-round moisture to flourish.

Where possible, choose land next to woodland, because it will retain moisture easily. Some commercial sources of Siberian Ginseng use pesticides and chemical fertilizers, so choose plants that have been grown with organic fertilizers only and no pesticides.

LEFT **Siberian Ginseng** thrives in soil that is rich in leaf mold.

ORGANIC GINSENG

In Britain, the Soil Association monitors requests for organic certificates. To qualify, soil must have been free of chemicals and pesticides for at least two years. The European Community countries have a similar approach, so that organic herbs and food can be freely interchanged. The US is trying to develop a similar system, but it is not as uniformly organized, and laws vary from state to state. They do, however, have a prolific network of outlets available to the public.

GINSENG TEA

You can buy Siberian Ginseng root, fresh and dried, but the leaves are not usually available. Try growing your own (see pages 26–27) and using the leaves to make Ginseng tea.

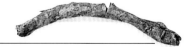

A history of healing

ALTHOUGH SIBERIAN GINSENG *is an ancient herb, widespread in the East, it was only classified botanically in the mid-19th century.*

TRADITIONAL USES

Siberian Ginseng has been used in Chinese and Asian traditional herbal medicine for over 2,000 years, and can be traced back much further in many ancient herbals. These herbals suggest that it has been known for as long as 5,000 years.

In a great Chinese book called the *Pen Ts'aos*, which represents over 4,000 years of Chinese medical knowledge, Siberian

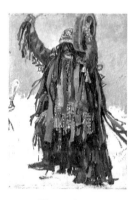

ABOVE *Siberian shamans have always considered herbs to be a vital ingredient in healing rituals.*

Ginseng was noted to be helpful for promoting energy and the treatment of rheumatism, and was used as a tonic. It was also used to treat sexual debility, lumbago, and excessive urination, as well as to strengthen the skeleton and tendons, and prevent ageing.

COMMON NAMES

The word "Ginseng" derives from the ancient Chinese *Jen Shen*, which means "man root." In 1900, Zaricor and Kweibin, two Chinese researchers, referred to it as *Chi Wu Cha* and *Wa Cha Seng*, but the most common name is *Ciwujia*. In Russia it is sometimes called the Free-berried Shrub. Other names include Wild Pepper, Russian Root, Devil's Bush, and Touch-me-not; the last two names no doubt refer to the plant's intimidating thorns!

Siberian Ginseng is often referred to as Eleuthero (a Latin abbreviation). It was also known by its now-obsolete Latin names *Acanthopanax senticosus*, *Hedera senticosa*, and *Aralia manchuria*.

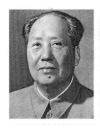

LEFT *Mao Zedong's reforms generated research into Siberian Ginseng.*

Russian botanist Carl Ivonovich Maximovich "discovered" Siberian Ginseng in 1854 in a remote area in southeast Russia. Four years later, the Russians gave it its Latin name.

Chinese Communist Party leader Chairman Mao (1893–1976) furthered research into Siberian Ginseng by expressing a desire for Chinese traditional medicine to be fused with Western methods.

In 1959 the Ministry of Health in what was then the USSR authorized clinical tests, which sparked a huge interest from the scientific community and the public. The Soviet Government then officially approved the herb's use as a tonic stimulant, and commercial production of the plant followed. Olympic athletes, miners, divers,

GINSENG'S REVIVAL

With the world evolving at a faster pace, humans need adaptogenic herbs more than ever. The pace of modern life means that many of us can barely keep up, and while this can encourage a stimulating lifestyle, it is all too often an exhausting process. The ability of Siberian Ginseng to help us deal with stress, physically and emotionally, has led to its current popularity; in particular, it helps our immune systems cope with the constant stream of pollutants encountered in everyday life.

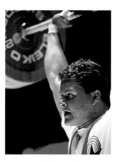

ABOVE *Siberian Ginseng was popular with athletes for improving stamina.*

climbers, soldiers, mountain rescuers, explorers, and cosmonauts began to use Siberian Ginseng. All this use and information was made possible by Professor Brekhman, the foremost recognized scientist and writer on this plant in former Soviet Russia.

As a result, Siberian Ginseng has been officially recognized and used by the Russian Government and its people for more than 30 years.

To date, over 1,000 articles have been published worldwide about Siberian Ginseng.

Anatomy of Siberian Ginseng

WHILE BOTH THE roots and leaves of Siberian Ginseng can be used in the preparation of remedies, the roots and rhizomes of this plant tend to dominate the commercial market.

LEFT **The bright green leaves are similar to horse chestnut.**

ROOTS

Siberian Ginseng roots are thick at the top, but they soon spread and turn into rhizomes that extend across the soil rather than going down into it. This usually happens in leaf mold and humus-rich woodland soil, and the growth eventually becomes profuse and webbed. Though each rhizome is quite thin, approximately ⅗in (1.5cm) in width, and only thickens a little at the base, it is in general round, woody, and pliable.

SHELF LIFE OF ROOTS
dried whole root lasts 1–2 years; dried root, cut or shredded, lasts about a year; powdered root lasts 6 months; fresh root lasts 2 weeks.

LEAVES

The leaves are used less than the roots, but are invaluable because they can be harvested and used medicinally while leaving the mother plant intact. They are bright green and borne on a long stalk in groups of three, four, or five small leaves about 5–6in (14cm) long. The leaves have two types of underside: one is smooth, the other is covered with short, fine, brown "fur." They can also grow in Europe in humus-rich, moist soil.

SHELF LIFE OF LEAVES
whole leaf lasts 6–12 months; shredded leaf lasts 6–9 months.

Chemical constituents

The chemistry of Siberian Ginseng is complex, and while it remains much the same in the root as in the leaf, the root is a little more potent. The main chemical impact is due to the plant's glycosides, which are often called eleutherosides; sixteen are known to date. There are also six senticosides (see page 57). These chemical compounds are responsible for a range of hormonal and immune system activities and act as plant steroids that support and fuel the adrenal glands.

Siberian Ginseng also has many other chemical components, which instigate hormonal activity and other basic processes.

RESPIRATORY AND DIGESTIVE SYSTEM

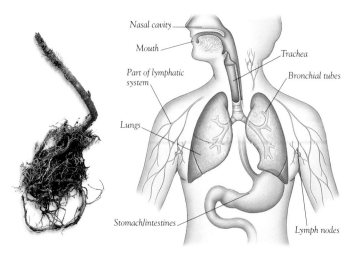

Nasal cavity

Mouth

Part of lymphatic system

Lungs

Stomach/intestines

Trachea

Bronchial tubes

Lymph nodes

ABOVE *The root's chemical constituents are more potent than those in the leaves.*

ABOVE *Siberian Ginseng regulates hormones and invigorates the immune system.*

Siberian Ginseng in action

SIBERIAN GINSENG IS *special because it balances all the many different types of cells in the body and therefore has an impressively wide and diverse range of positive effects on the body and its wellbeing.*

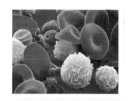

RIGHT **Ginseng energizes blood cells and helps them to fight infection.**

HOW SIBERIAN GINSENG CAN HELP

Siberian Ginseng is a stimulating tonic. In this context, "stimulating" means the ability to increase the work capacity of the entire body after only a single dose. The tonic effect maintains its impact over a prolonged period of time, keeping the energies revitalised without overworking the body. It even continues working for a period of time *after* you have stopped taking it.

RIGHT **All types of Ginseng have tonic benefits.**

Herb stimulants that are not equally balanced with toning effects can be destructive, ultimately diminishing output and even becoming detrimental to health: happily, this is not a problem with Siberian Ginseng.

CAUTION

The powerful *Ren shen* (Red Ginseng) can also quickly make a person feel energized and revived, but if the body is weak and depleted, *Ren shen* will ultimately make things worse – even to the point of collapse. Siberian is the safest and most effective Ginseng, and in 20 years of using it, the author has never come across any unpleasant side effects or adverse reactions.

ADAPTOGENIC HERB

Siberian Ginseng is known as an adaptogen because it heals and energizes the whole body without any unpleasant side effects. The term was introduced (because of this herb and subsequently others) by the Russian Professor A. P. Golikov. He suggested that an adaptogenic herb should meet three criteria, and cited Siberian Ginseng to set the standard:

1. Produces an overall normalizing action on the body, irrespective of any particular illness or unbalanced state.
2. Produces a non-specific but positive action that ultimately increases resistance to a range of potentially adverse influences, whether these influences are of a physical, chemical, or biochemical nature.
3. Causes no side effects – or at least only minimal disorder – in the physiological functioning of a human being or animal.

STRESS AND SIBERIAN GINSENG

Stress detrimentally involves a number of organs and systems – neurotransmitters, neuromodulators, hormones, the immune system, and adrenal glands. However, stress levels are individual, and levels of adrenal function are often genetically predetermined. Our ability to adapt to situations is therefore also genetic. If this variable

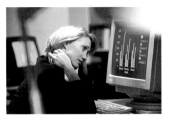

ABOVE *The negative effects of stress can be lessened with Siberian Ginseng.*

capacity is used up, the adrenal glands enlarge, the thymus gland becomes unbalanced, and the immune system plummets.

Siberian Ginseng helps us to accept a range of adverse circumstances by balancing the alarm reaction of the adrenal glands, nervous system, and other related areas of the body, a response that can be mild, moderate, or so severe that it may eventually lead to serious illness. Sometimes stress simply continues at a relentless (if not life-threatening) pace, but should long-term exposure to stress continue, the body can become totally exhausted and even collapse under the pressure. Siberian Ginseng will support the body if it is introduced at this stage or can even prevent this stage from being reached if taken in time.

HOW SIBERIAN GINSENG AFFECTS THE BODY

Siberian Ginseng has many valuable properties, including:

❋ Antidiuretic (prevents excessive release of water from the body).

❋ Antiedemic (prevents retention of water in the body).

❋ Antioxidant (protects the body's cells from damage by free radicals – see page 55).

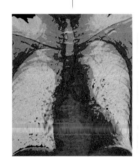

RIGHT *The overall health of the lungs is improved because the herb increases oxygen intake.*

EFFECTS

❋ Increases the body's ability to resist infection.

❋ Helps to prevent cardiac pains, and pains in and around the neck and head such as headache.

❋ Aids nerve centers and message conduction to the brain.

❋ Improves cerebral corticoid (steroid hormone) function and the speed of the brain.

❋ Alleviates neurodynamic disturbance, and neurological movement and growth, by helping neurotransmitters to function efficiently.

❋ Enhances liver protection and lessens liver cell degeneration.

❋ Increases semen output and heightens both male and female fertility.

❋ Increases oxygen consumption and improves respiratory effectiveness.

❋ Breaks down and clears the body of drug residues.

❋ Helps the body resist and may even prevent tuberculosis.

❋ Assists the body to maintain cellular homeostasis.

❋ Helps the treatment of skin inflammations, dandruff, acne, hair falling out, and all general skin and hair problems.

❋ Aids the brain by helping neurological pathways to work better; useful for dyslexia, autism, cranial cerebral injury, fits, epilepsy, and general memory retention.

❋ Improves hearing and sight.

❋ Helps prevent ageing.

SIBERIAN GINSENG IN THE BODY

The herb works effectively at many different levels in the body and assists the various body systems to function efficiently

Brain	Hair
Hearing	Sight
Metabolism	Thymus
Arteries	Heart
Lungs	Spleen
Blood	Liver
Muscles	Nervous system
Skin	Fertility
Immune system	Cell homeostasis

RIGHT *Siberian Ginseng promotes a wealth of positive responses in body systems.*

GINSENG AND THE BLOOD

Siberian Ginseng is able to produce a profound effect on the blood. It can:

* Balance blood pressure (but it is not recommended for people with a reading of 180/90mmHg or higher – see page 21).

* Reduce cholesterol and triglyceride levels (see page 57)

* Normalize blood protein levels.

* Help balance blood sugar levels.

* Positively influence RNA synthesis (see page 57).

* Restore hemoglobin levels in cases of blood loss.

* Normalize arterial pressure, increase arterial wall elasticity, and help treat hardening of the arteries, including arteriosclerosis.

* Prevent too many white blood cells from developing.

* Normalize circulation or cerebral hemodynamics (the dynamics of blood movement).

BELOW **Siberian Ginseng boosts blood-vessel health.**

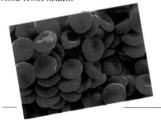

ANTI-INFLAMMATORY AGENT

Siberian Ginseng is noted for its anti-inflammatory properties. When the immune system is no longer capable of working in a balanced way, it goes into overdrive and produces a variety of counterproductive symptoms and side effects. While a little inflammation protects damaged tissue, an excessive amount impedes the healing process, blocking adequate circulation and the passage of nutritional components.

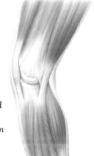

RIGHT **The painful inflammation of a strained muscle can be soothed by Siberian Ginseng.**

BLOOD SUGAR LEVELS

Siberian Ginseng helps diabetics and hypoglycemics, partly by lowering serum glucose levels. It aids the resynthesis of glycogen and high energy phosphorus compounds, and daily excretion of sugar is drastically reduced. It also prevents an increase of adrenal function, which goes into action to counter stress when glucose cannot be retained.

GINSENG AND THE MIND

In cases of neurosis, chronic abnormal fatigue, hysteria, depression, loss of appetite, moderate depression, inability to concentrate, insomnia, and psychosis, Siberian Ginseng is able to stimulate and activate inhibitory processes as required, thus re-establishing balance. It allows more concentration, less depression, and better sleep.

GINSENG AND AFTERCARE

Siberian Ginseng can be used in various postoperative forms to:

⚹ Assist recovery from chronic illness.

⚹ Reduce weight gain of thymus and spleen following cortisone medication.

⚹ Decrease adverse reactions to vaccines and antibiotics.

CAUTION

Current investigation into the chemical composition of Siberian Ginseng suggests that it might not be appropriate for people with very high arterial blood pressure, so consult your doctor first.

GINSENG AND EVERYDAY PROBLEMS

Siberian Ginseng increases resistance to any negative, stress-induced reactions – physically, chemically, biologically, and psychologically. It reduces irritability, aids work capacity, lessens neurotic behavior, and alleviates general anxiety.

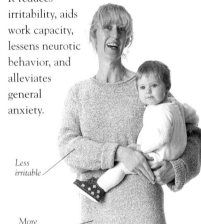

Less irritable

More relaxed

Better able to cope

RIGHT **Children can sap energy levels, but Siberian Ginseng helps to restore balance.**

OTHER EFFECTS

Siberian Ginseng increases anabolic activity and carbohydrate and protein metabolism, producing an increase in strength and endurance and providing protection against hypothermia. The herb is therefore very useful for divers, climbers, mountain rescuers, soldiers, explorers,

RADIATION AND TOXINS

Siberian Ginseng helps protect against radiation and was used in the aftermath of the Chernobyl disaster in the Ukraine in the 1980s. It generally helps reduce the toxic effects of chemicals and increases the absorption of food, vitamins, and minerals.

and even cosmonauts. It also counteracts the effects of sore muscles after muscular activity so it is good for all types of athletic activity.

Siberian Ginseng's reputation for aiding male sexuality has made it a traditional favorite with older men in the East and recently in the West. Its claims to fame include stronger sex drive, increased semen output, and heightened fertility – all accomplished without decreasing energy levels at any point. But it is no male preserve: the herb also helps women to become more sexually active and fertile.

RIGHT *The herb helps the body work efficiently in harsh conditions.*

CASE STUDY: FLU

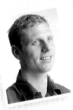

Tom had a bout of flu and took a long time to recover. A 29-year-old manager in a busy firm, he suffered two months of fatigue. At the end of each day, he felt worse; even if he was getting ready to go out, he would suddenly feel exhausted, shivery, and weak, and lose his appetite.

A herbalist, recommended by a friend, prescribed a program of good food, plenty of rest, moderate exercise, and initially high doses of Siberian Ginseng. After two weeks on 1 tsp (5ml) of tincture five times a day, he felt his old self returning: he had more energy and no longer experienced the evening symptoms. He felt stronger, more lively, and more interested in life.

The herbalist then lowered the dose to 1 tsp (5ml) three times a day, and within weeks Tom had bounced back to a complete recovery.

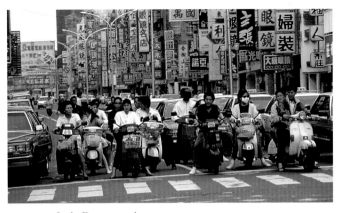

ABOVE **In the East, men and women still trust Siberian Ginseng to increase their sexual potency and fertility.**

The claims for Siberian Ginseng are not exaggerated – this herb really is known as the "King of Adaptogens." But it is usually seen more in terms of background support and is often added to patients' herb programs, especially if they show signs of tiredness, immune system deficiency, hormonal complications, nervous system weakness, or stress. Siberian Ginseng is the perfect tonic to help all of us in today's hectic world, and can be complemented by other good food and helpful herbs.

WHEN TO AVOID SIBERIAN GINSENG

This herb is one of the least toxic herbal agents known. However, Professor A.P. Golikov suggested in the 1960s that Siberian Ginseng should not be used for some problems, including tachycardia, extrasystole (heart B. peval), hypertonicity, high arterial blood pressure, and certain types of insomnia (see pages 56–57). As yet, no evidence has been found to support this theory, and at the time minor side effects were found in only two out of 1,000 studies. These may have had other causes: in the authors' long experience, and that of many colleagues, there has never been a case of adverse reaction to this herb.

Energy and emotion

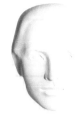

SIBERIAN GINSENG CAN *help strengthen the mind via its positive effects on the physical body. It boosts stamina and encourages a real zest for life. It can*

LEFT **Siberian Ginseng encourages a positive approach to life.**

also enable you to clarify your thoughts and become more decisive and better balanced emotionally.

Siberian Ginseng is bitter-sweet, with a warming, acrid flavor. This taste strongly supports the basic energy and strength of the body. According to traditional Chinese medicine, it enters primarily through the kidneys and secondarily via the spleen, pancreas, and liver. People who lack energy in these organs may sometimes feel like being alone and may not wish to relate to people; they can also have a fear of the cold and feel timid and exhausted. Siberian Ginseng's flavors can help to change some of these distressing mental states and treat a wide variety of physical symptoms.

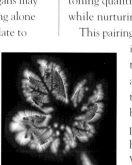

ABOVE **Kirlian photography enables us to see the spirit energy of a plant.**

In the West, bitter flavors traditionally sharpen and tone appetite. Bitter herbs encourage the digestive system to work more efficiently. When the sweet and bitter tastes are combined, the result is a harmonious union of taste, which brings in supportive and toning qualities that energize while nurturing.

This pairing of flavors takes into account that the individual is already tired and that on its own the bitter flavor could prove to be too harsh a taskmaster. When combined, however, these two flavors stimulate the body while building and healing.

SCHIZOPHRENIA

Scientific evidence from the 1950s proved that many schizophrenic patients suffered from very low adrenal function (adrenal burnout), probably genetically inherited.

Schizophrenia is an illness of the body as well as the mind inasmuch as organs and systems can create body chemistry that adversely affects the mind. Siberian Ginseng can help in the treatment of schizophrenia by alleviating some of the stress and negative emotions associated with this condition.

ENERGY AND THE MIND

Through its taste, energy, and chemistry, Siberian Ginseng can make a huge difference to your thoughts, feelings, and actions via the adrenals, kidneys, liver, stomach, pancreas, and spleen, and create a positive chain reaction in the mind. Taking Siberian Ginseng can sometimes feel like wearing glasses after being nearsighted for a long time. Unhappiness and fatigue can slip away, and a zest for life – either missing for a long period or never felt at all – can become apparent.

PERSONAL GROWTH

Any form of stress or crisis, with or without long-term exhaustion, can create negative chain reactions. If these are allowed to remain and fester, they can produce bitterness, defeatism, "victim" states of mind, fearfulness, and a lack of confidence. Stress and crisis situations also create the possibility that there will be less love to go around (for yourself as well as others) because of the emotionally exhausting negative chain reactions they induce.

Siberian Ginseng can support and energize you both physically and mentally. It can help in situations that are noncritical but where life may lack excitement. Its far-reaching chemistries tone the hormone system, support all the major organs, trigger positive immune-system reactions, and balance the nervous system and the mind.

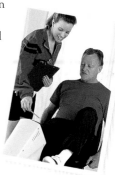

ABOVE *Use Siberian Ginseng to keep mind and body in peak condition.*

FLOWER REMEDIES

When in flower, Siberian Ginseng provides a striking and beautiful sight. Its cream or pastel colored umbrellas of starlike clusters punctuate the darkness of the woodlands it inhabits. It is as if little moons are radiating in the forest and whispering their gifts of harmony, balance, and sanity. For those individuals who have a tendency to float off mentally like passing clouds, or who find it hard to think, remember, or focus, this remedy will solidify and "ground" them. For all of us, this flower remedy can help to illuminate our thoughts and balance our emotions.

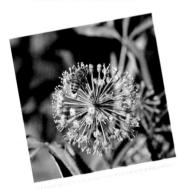

ABOVE **Ginseng's starry flowers can be distilled into a harmonizing tonic.**

TO MAKE A FLOWER ESSENCE

STANDARD QUANTITY

Approx. 1½ cups (350ml) each of spring water and brandy, and 3–4 Siberian Ginseng flowers.

1 *Submerge carefully chosen, freshly picked flowers in a glass bowl of spring water. Cover with clean white cheesecloth and put in the sunshine for at least three hours. If the flowers wilt sooner, remove them earlier.*

2 *Use a twig to lift the flowers from the bowl. Measure the remaining liquid, add an equal amount of brandy, then pour into dark glass bottles. Label clearly.*

Recommended dosage

Adults: 4 drops under the tongue 4 times daily, or every half hour in times of crisis. Children: over 12 years, adult dose; 7–12 years, ½ adult dose; 1–7 years, ¼ adult dose; younger than 1, consult a herbalist.

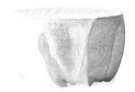

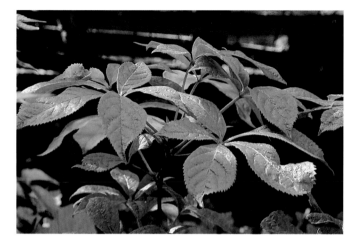

PLANT SPIRIT ENERGIES

This shrub inhabits the "middle height" in the canopies of woods and forests: it neither stays close to the ground nor reaches the tops of the trees. It grows in harmony with all that surrounds it, giving and receiving shade and nutrition. Siberian Ginseng is a great survivor, and as a young plant, its thorns protect it and keep predators away while its procreative abilities enable it to diversify and survive.

Adaptive, creative, and beautiful, Siberian Ginseng has a spirit that wants to survive and achieve, but not at the expense of its own or the energy of others. It shares its gifts with a generous spirit. This particular spirit is much needed, given the various environmental problems now facing the earth and its inhabitants.

Siberian Ginseng can help us all to adapt and can give us the strength and endurance to meet everyday obstacles. Meeting these problems with enthusiasm will help the solutions to be more creative and positive.

ABOVE *Siberian Ginseng adapts to its environment; taking the herb confers adaptogenic qualities.*

Growing, harvesting, and processing

WHETHER YOU DECIDE to grow your own from seed or purchase a seedling from a commercial source, Siberian Ginseng is easy to cultivate and worth the effort because it can be put to a variety of uses.

ABOVE *You will need soil rich in leaf mold to grow Ginseng.*

GROWING SIBERIAN GINSENG

Although it is a long process, there should be no problems growing your own Siberian Ginseng as long as the soil is loam-based, rich in humus (leaf mold) – with a little grit if you mix your own – and has a good moisture content. While this shrub cannot tolerate relentless heat that dries out its roots, it will grow well in full sun if it is always kept moist.

Plants growing in the sun will produce a lot of top foliage and reach heights of 10ft (3m) in 10–15 years, but they may reach only 3ft (1m) in the same time if grown in shaded conditions, where they will instead produce more roots. Woodland clearings are suitable for planting a small grove, but growing a single plant in a tiny backyard is equally feasible. Make sure you keep the plants well watered, especially in full sun.

You can either purchase a seedling or young plant from a nursery, or germinate your own

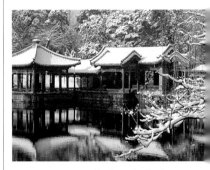

ABOVE *Seed germination is a slow process and requires frosty conditions for success.*

from seed. The key to successful germination is to bear in mind the plant's cold origins: it needs frost to mobilize its procreativity.

Put seeds in a clay pot with a suitable soil mix and leave outside for 18 months with only a glass covering in order to break their dormancy. In the colder parts of Europe and North America, this process is only necessary for 6–12 months in order to break dormancy.

1. The soil mix in the clay pot should be a mixture of good-quality loam, leaf mold, and grit.

2. Bury a few seeds in the soil, halfway up the pot. Cover with soil to within 1" (2.5cm) of the pot's rim to allow for watering.

3. Bury the pot in sand up to the rim. Cover with a sheet of glass.

Ideally, this should be done in October or November – giving it the following winter, summer, and second winter in this state. The following spring should give rise to an emerging seedling.

Once they are large enough, repot the seedlings or plant them out in a seedling bed.

The nurseryman who provides the seed will himself have collected the whole black berries in October. He will have dried and then rubbed them to reveal the individual seeds. You will eventually be able to collect your own seeds in this way.

ABOVE After planting seeds, you should bury the pot in sand.

If planting out bought or self-germinated seedlings, you will need to provide exactly the right soil and moisture requirements. Repeat the soil mix of loam, leaf mold, and grit each winter to renew the ability to retain water and nutrients.

LEFT Water your plant copiously and regularly.

GINSENG ROOT

Digging up your Ginseng root would be a shame and is not necessary. Instead harvest the leaves and purchase the root.

HARVESTING

Harvesting takes place in field-grown situations or in the wild in woodlands and forests. Some leaves and large amounts of the rhizome are harvested at their peak. In the case of leaves, this is when they unfurl during the spring and summer.

Harvesting continues throughout the season as long as enough plants are left to ensure their continuation. Roots and rhizomes are harvested in October, but timing varies from area to area. The determining factor is when the top foliage has begun to die, indicating that growth has ceased for the season.

Plants grown in shaded or woodland conditions produce less top growth and more root; the opposite is true if they grow in open fields. When the shrubs are at least five years old, the roots are lifted from the soil either using machinery or by hand using a five-pronged fork. No harm must come to the roots in any way. Once raised, the roots are collected and kept in a cool, shady spot until they can be processed, preferably on the same day.

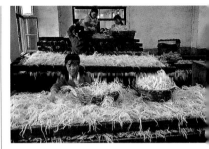

ABOVE *The crop is harvested from spring to summer, then sorted, cleaned, and dried.*

Harvesting the leaves can be done at any time during the spring and summer. There will be small variations in chemistries, with spring leaves slightly more potent, but these differences are almost insignificant. Use the leaves as fresh as possible, either chewing them or brewing them as a tea.

To dry the leaves for winter use, lay them on drying racks or cake racks, above a stove or radiator, or place a few in paper bags and suspend them from string in the driest room you have available.

Turn and shake the leaves regularly to prevent spoiling and to keep moisture from collecting. Put a few leaves in a glass jar, tighten the lid, and place it in full sun; if droplets of water appear, reprocess the leaves until they are completely dry.

PROCESSING

Within a few hours of digging up the roots, lay them out on wooden or wire table screens and then spray them with water or submerge them in tubs. Either way, dirt clinging to the roots needs to be loosened without the force of the water harming the skin. You do not have to clean off every last speck of dirt. It is actually better to leave the skin of the root intact and dirty rather than lacerated and open to microbial invasion.

After washing, lay the roots in the shade to drain for a couple of hours before drying begins. Because wet roots will eventually start to rot, air drying must follow draining. While large roots can take up to six weeks to dry out, smaller ones may take only a few days. Air temperature is vital, so use a well-insulated room with good heat retention. Electricity, wood, gas, and oil can all be employed to generate the heat needed.

Do not dry the outside of the root too quickly – this will cause hardening while still leaving the inside moist. The room temperature should be kept at around 70°F (19.5°C), though this may be raised slightly after a few days. Check closely for signs of excess moisture returning and spoilage by mildew.

Both overheating and cool temperatures are the enemy of drying out roots successfully. The sign of properly and thoroughly dried roots is that they will not bend but will break with a clean "snap." They will then be ready to store in dry, well-ventilated conditions in wooden or thick cardboard containers.

It is important that the roots do not reabsorb water by being stored in the wrong conditions. For export, they are often packed into woven burlap bags, labeled, and then sent as quickly as possible to their destination.

RIGHT **Roots must be stored in dry conditions to avoid absorbing damp.**

Preparations for internal use

WHETHER YOU USE root or leaf, Siberian Ginseng is confined to internal use. The choice is wide: tincture, decoction, infusion, wine, soup, tablets, and capsules.

LEFT *Choose fresh Siberian* **Ginseng wherever possible, but dried can be used if necessary.**

TINCTURE

This is an excellent way of extracting the medicinal effects of Siberian Ginseng. If you buy it ready-made from a supplier, a tincture requires no further preparation and can be kept for up to three years.

Siberian Ginseng tincture is made by soaking the pre-chopped or shredded root, root rind (or bark), and rhizomes in alcohol and water. You can also use powdered root, but it must be fresh quality because powders in general deteriorate much more quickly than the shredded root.

Alcohol is poured onto the roots in order to kill any germs, and the water is added two days later, once any undesirable microbes are dead.

Commercially, Siberian Ginseng tincture is made with good-quality, high-percentage 80% proof alcohol with a combination of 45% alcohol and 55% water. Homemade tinctures have the advantage of your personal handling and care.

Tinctures are often made at the new moon, and strained and bottled at the full moon.

NOTE

Always use utensils cleaned in boiling water – and for good results add one or two drops of lavender, thyme, or tea-tree essential oil to the water.

TO MAKE A TINCTURE

STANDARD QUANTITY

Use 8oz (225g) of dried roots or 11oz (310g) of fresh roots,
chopped into small pieces or bought shredded, added to
4 cups (1 liter) of alcohol and water mixture

1 *Put the fresh or dried Siberian Ginseng roots and rhizomes into a liquidizer and cover with vodka; 45% proof is standard, but 70–80% proof is better. Liquidize the ingredients – the mixture will be stiff and hard, but persist. Pour the mixture into a large dark glass jar. Cover with an airtight lid. Shake well, label the jar carefully, and store in a dark place.*

2 *After two days, measure the contents and add water – add 20% water if using standard vodka and 50–60% water if using 70–80% proof vodka. The whole tincturing process will take at least 14 days, but you can leave it for up to four weeks. Remember to shake the jar daily to aid the extraction process.*

3 *Strain the tincture through a jelly-bag, preferably overnight, until you have the very last drop. For best results you can use a wine press.*

4 *Pour the thick liquid into dark jars and label clearly. Store in a cool, dark place. For personal use, decant into a 2fl oz (50ml) tincture bottle.*

For dosages, see page 32.

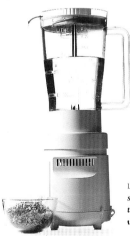

LEFT **It will take
some time to liquidize
the chopped root and
vodka mixture.**

RECOMMENDED DOSAGES
FOR TINCTURES

🌿 **Everyday use** *The adult standard dose is 1–2 tsp (5–10ml) twice daily, diluted in approximately 5 tsp (25ml) of water or fruit juice. When you are trying to resolve a situation rapidly, use a total of 4–8 tsp (20–40ml) per day. This can be reduced to 1 tsp (5ml) 3 times daily, a total of 3 tsp (15ml) per day once the condition is calmer and symptoms are less severe. Long-term support is then the aim (see below).*

🌿 **Long-term use** *Adults can take 1–2 tsp (5–10ml) daily for 6–9 months, and it will continue to exert its beneficial effects for a few months after this point. It may be necessary to begin use again after a break should stress levels remain high, perhaps over years rather than months. Resuming in this way is perfectly acceptable and can protect the body from long-term damage and stress.*

🌿 **Children's dosages** *Over 12 years, 1–2 tsp (5–10 ml) twice daily; 9–12 years, 30 drops 1–3 times daily; 1–9 years, 5 drops 2–3 times daily; younger than 1, 2 drops twice daily.*

ROOT QUALITY

Fresh Ginseng root is always the best choice, although it may be hard to obtain except for those close to an available source, for example Japan, Mongolia, China, or Russia. However, good-quality, well-harvested, and carefully dried roots also make excellent quality medicines.

REMOVING
THE ALCOHOL

Diabetics, hypoglycemics, and pregnant women may not wish to imbibe the small amount of alcohol contained in the tincture. Therefore add a little boiling water to your dose and leave to stand for five minutes while evaporation takes place; roughly 98.5% of the alcohol will evaporate. For non-drinkers, tinctures can also be made using apple cider vinegar instead of alcohol – although bear in mind that the extraction of the beneficial chemical content will not be as complete without the use of alcohol.

LEFT *Siberian Ginseng root is safe to chew and makes an excellent medicine.*

DECOCTION

This is an ideal way to prepare the root and seed of Siberian Ginseng. Fresh or dried root and seed may be used, although fresh is always the best choice. Decoctions preserve all the qualities and chemical components of Siberian Ginseng very efficiently.

It is best to make the decoction fresh each day, although you can make it in bulk quantities if time is short. You can keep the decoction in the refrigerator for up to three days, but no longer.

TO MAKE A DECOCTION

STANDARD QUANTITY

¾oz (20g) dried roots or 1½oz (40g) chopped or shredded fresh roots to 3 cups (750ml) cold water, reduced to about 2 cups (500ml) after simmering

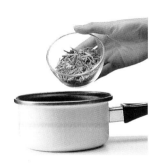

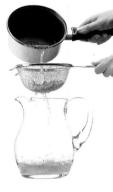

2 Let the liquid cool and then strain it into a pitcher, keeping a little aside for your first cup. Put the remainder in a cool place, or refrigerate it if you are going to store the decoction for longer than a day.

1 Place the chopped or shredded roots with the water in a saucepan (a double boiler is ideal). Bring to a boil, and then simmer on a low heat for about 20–30 minutes. The liquid should reduce by about one third. Remove the pan from the heat.

Recommended dosage
*Adults: 2 cups (500ml) daily.
Children: over 12 years, adult dose; 9–12 years, half adult dose; 1–9 years, quarter adult dose; younger than 1, 1 tsp (5ml) 1–2 times daily.*

INFUSION

While the roots are better extracted in water using a decoction or simmering process, making Siberian Ginseng leaf tea from your own plants is an ideal and very popular way of using the plant's leaves, and is a useful way of taking this herb to maintain general good health.

TO MAKE AN INFUSION

STANDARD QUANTITY

1 tsp (2–3g) of crumbled, dried leaf or
2 tsp (4–6g) of fresh chopped leaf, to 1 cup (250ml) of boiling water

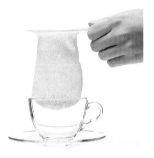

Recommended dosage

Adults: 2 cups (500ml) daily for recovery from illness, or ½ cup (125ml) daily for general good health. Children: over 12, adult dose; 9–12, half adult dose; 1–9 quarter adult dose; younger than 1, 2 tsp (10ml) daily.

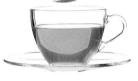

1 *Put the herb in a tea sock and place in a cup or teapot. Pour on the boiling water and leave to stand for 7 minutes.*

2 *Remove the tea sock and, if desired, add half a teaspoon of organic, cold pressed honey to the tea (although teas are usually best without added sweeteners).*

NOTE

Teas can also be made in a special teapot infuser, or in a coffeepot with a plunger.

CAPSULES

Capsules can be made simply by using commercially powdered Siberian Ginseng. Make sure you ask about the shelf life of the herb that you are buying: it should be no older than a year when you receive it, and preferably less than six months to insure maximum potency.

If you are a vegetarian, it will be better to choose casings from vegetable sources in preference to those of animal origin, although they tend to be more expensive.

The root should have a sweetly bitter flavor – not fierce in either direction but pleasantly harmonious and earthy. Any blandness means it is an old powder and should be returned, because this root in particular loses its saponin content (see page 57) a little after powdering. Capsules seal in the powder and prevent further loss, but powders do not last as long as whole, chopped, shredded, or crumbled herb, because the larger surface area is more exposed to oxygen and thus deterioration.

TO MAKE CAPSULES

STANDARD QUANTITY

Approx. 500–600mg of powdered herb fits into an average-size capsule

1 Put a little dried, finely powdered Siberian Ginseng in a saucer.

2 Open the capsule ends. Using the ends as shovels, push them together until they are full. Slide the capsule ends together carefully.

Recommended dosage
Adults: 2–3 capsules twice daily.
Children: over 12 years, adult dose; 9–12 years, 1–2 capsules twice daily; 5–9 years, 1 capsule twice daily; do not give to children younger than 5.

RIGHT **Dredge the capsule halves through the powder and push together.**

TABLETS

If you prefer tablets to capsules, you can make your own tablets quite simply by using finely powdered root. They should be made up just prior to use, but can be stored in the refrigerator for up to a day in airtight containers. You do not necessarily need to sweeten Siberian Ginseng because it has a very pleasing flavor of its own, which in itself stimulates beneficial digestive reactions.

CHEWING THE ROOT

A small piece of good-quality Siberian Ginseng root can be slowly chewed for 10–15 minutes 2–3 times a day. A piece the size of a baby's fingernail is adequate. Once all the flavor has disappeared, the resulting woody roughage can be discarded – or swallowed for useful fiber intake.

TO MAKE TABLETS

STANDARD QUANTITY

Use 2–4g finely powdered root to 5 or more drops of bottled water

Mix a little water with the powder and roll into tablets of convenient size. For added sweetness, you can add a little maple syrup or honey. The overall consistency should be like pastry.

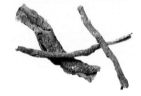

NOTE

When buying tablets, check with the manufacturer that there is as little additional material in the pill as possible in order to gain as much of the real root and leaf as you can.

Recommended dosage

Adults: 2–3 tablets twice daily. Children: over 12 years, adult dose; 9–12 years, 1–2 tablets twice daily; 5–9 years, 1 tablet twice daily; do not give to children younger than 5.

SIBERIAN GINSENG SOUP

This is a lovely way of giving medicine to people who are convalescing after illness. It can be cooked with other fortifying roots like yams, potatoes, and carrots, and seasoned with herbs and Shiitake mushrooms together with a little salt and garlic – all of which will further boost the immune system.

TO MAKE SIBERIAN GINSENG SOUP

INGREDIENTS

4–5 cups (1–1.25 liters) distilled or bottled water
1oz (25g) dried Siberian Ginseng root, shredded
1oz (25g) potato, yam, or carrots, chopped (or use two or all three)
handful of Shiitake mushrooms
1–2 garlic cloves
pinch of sea salt
fresh or dried thyme or marjoram, chopped, to taste

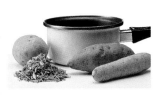

1 *Bring the water to a boil in a pan. Add the Siberian Ginseng and root vegetables and simmer for 20 minutes until they are soft.*

2 *Purée the liquid and the vegetables, then add the finely chopped mushrooms, garlic, salt, and herbs.*

3 *Warm the soup for a further 7–10 minutes on low heat, then serve.*

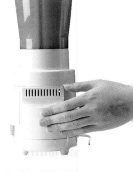

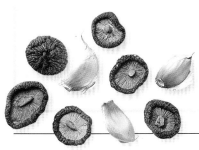

ROOT WINE

Root wine is an ancient Chinese treatment for the elderly. Old people who suffered from rheumatism would make and drink this wine on a daily basis, because it was as pleasant as medicine could get! It will help to reduce swelling, poor circulation, coldness, dampness, and other symptoms associated with rheumatism. It is an ideal remedy for those with long-term debilitation rather than those with acute conditions.

Home-brewing and wine-making suppliers can provide the yeast culture and necessary equipment for you to make your own Siberian Ginseng wine. You will need to buy sterilizing tablets to make sure all the equipment is clean – this is of

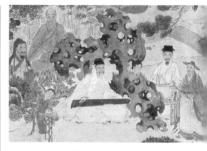

ABOVE *Tonic wines were traditionally used by the Chinese for convalescence.*

paramount importance because contamination can easily result in a spoiled brew.

The wine is made by first making a tea, dissolving sugar or honey into it, and then, when it is cold, adding live yeast culture. This slowly ferments, and when the fermentation is almost complete, the brew is strained and bottled.

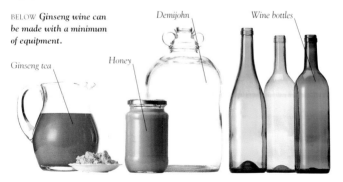

BELOW **Ginseng wine can be made with a minimum of equipment.**

Demijohn

Wine bottles

Honey

Ginseng tea

TO MAKE GINSENG WINE

STANDARD QUANTITY

5–9 pints (2.25–4.5 litres) of Siberian Ginseng tea
3–5lb (1.5–2.5kg) organic sugar
1 sachet of wine-making yeast (follow instructions on pack)

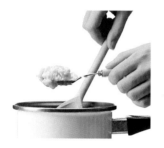

1 Mix the tea with sugar or honey by warming the tea in a saucepan and then stirring in sugar until it is completely dissolved.

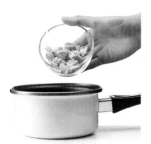

2 Remove from the heat, let it cool to about 65°F (18°C), then add the yeast.

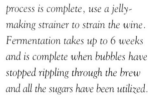

3 Let it ferment in a wine demijohn with a suitable neck lock so the carbon dioxide can escape freely.

4 When the fermentation process is complete, use a jelly-making strainer to strain the wine. Fermentation takes up to 6 weeks and is complete when bubbles have stopped rippling through the brew and all the sugars have been utilized.

5 Bottle the wine, label it clearly, then store it in cool conditions.

NOTE

Hurried and incomplete fermentation will produce an unpleasant wine. While fermentation is taking place, the demijohn should be left in a warm but shaded area.

Natural medicine for everyone

UNLIKE OTHER SPECIES of Ginseng, Siberian is believed to be *completely safe for most people, even those groups in society who are considered to be most vulnerable, such as pregnant women, children, invalids, and the elderly.*

PREGNANCY

Siberian Ginseng is renowned for encouraging better fertility in both men and women, and it is a wonderful herb for use during pregnancy because it maintains energy, reduces stress, and assists the balanced working of all organs and systems. It will also work safely instead of antibiotics to support the body through any microbial invasion.

Research in Russia has proved that the herb helped reduce neonatal disorders, especially newborn infants with defects in introcranial blood circulation. The incidence of stillborn babies also appeared to be lower in the trials. It has also been used successfully as an antibiotic agent for young babies. It encourages milk production too, resulting in calmer, happier breastfeeding mothers and their babies.

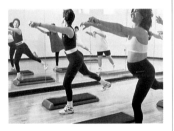

ABOVE *Ginseng tops up energy levels during pregnancy.*

CAUTION

Siberian Ginseng supports mothers-to-be, but it is vital that the correct herb is taken. Other Ginseng varieties can be dangerous, so:
- purchase the root from a reputable supplier
- ask for Siberian Ginseng
- check its Latin family name: *Eleutherococcus senticosus*

CHILDREN

Children benefit from Siberian Ginseng because it helps form brain components, helping them to become more alert and able to concentrate more effectively. It is also good for children who are hyperactive or who have memory or learning difficulties. It makes a wonderful remedy for many minor ailments, physical or mental. Low-weight children have successfully gained weight with Siberian Ginseng, and good general development has followed. Siberian Ginseng will help children of all ages play, rest, and work in a more balanced way, regulating and helping both physical and mental growth.

RIGHT
Children's concentration and memory are improved.

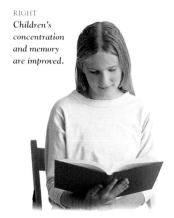

ELDERLY PEOPLE

Siberian Ginseng is particularly suitable for older people because of its ability to help a wide variety of problems associated with advancing age or even senility:

※ Increases self-confidence and alleviates depression.

※ Helps to maintain the brain and its blood supply, and aids memory.

※ Encourages sound sleep and generally strengthens the body, enabling the elderly to feel more physically capable.

※ Is a natural antioxidant that can slow down the effects of the aging process in older people.

CASE STUDY: ENERGY

Rosemary, 63, felt that her energy levels were waning fast – and she wished they would return. A chance conversation with a friend led her to start taking Siberian Ginseng bought from a herb shop. After ten days of taking just 1 tsp (5ml) of tincture twice a day, she noticed a growing difference in her overall energy levels. This led to a renewed zest for life and unprecedented patience with previously frustrating everyday situations.

Herbal combinations

HERBAL COMBINATIONS ARE *used where the effect of a single herb needs to be complemented in a particular way. However, if you are pregnant, breastfeeding, or have a serious medical condition, you should consult your doctor or another qualified medical practitioner because some of these herbs may be unsuitable.*

ANTISTRESS FORMULA

This herbal combination used as a tincture helps to build energy and specifically aims to put back the building blocks required by the adrenal glands, which are usually in short supply during times of stress.

Formula 3 parts Siberian Ginseng root, 2 parts Chamomile flowers, 2 parts Saw Palmetto berries, 2 parts St. John's Wort flowers and leaves, 2 parts Rehmannia root, 1 part Wild Yam rhizome.

Dosage Adults: 1 tsp (5ml) 3–4 times daily. Children: you should consult your doctor or a qualified herbalist.

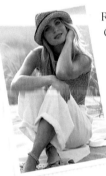

ABOVE **Anti-stress formula peps up depleted energy.**

Saw Palmetto, Rehmannia, Siberian Ginseng, and Wild Yam help the adrenal glands.

St. John's Wort supports the mind and helps to raise "happy hormone" levels. Chamomile supports a run-down nervous system.

CAUTION

The antistress formula must not be taken during pregnancy. Also, individuals taking drugs for depression or other mental disorders, or those with light sensitivity, should omit St. John's Wort from the herbal formula.

AUTOIMMUNE FORMULA

The immune system is not just part of our defense and healing team: it affects many systems in the body, and a poorly functioning immune system will affect our hormones, nervous system, and much more. The herbs in this formula, which should be taken as a tincture, aim to restore, tone, and balance the organs and body systems while motivating a positive and focused response from the immune system.

Autoimmune conditions arise out of an "all systems down" situation, where the body is so low that it works on overdrive. This formula avoids herbs that overstimulate the immune system even more and instead focuses on gentle and broadly based immune-system herbs, producing a climate in which the immune system may be able to recognize that it does not need to work in overdrive, yet at the same time empowering it.

Formula 3 parts Siberian Ginseng root, 2 parts Burdock root, 2 parts Schisandra berries, 2 parts Marshmallow root, ¼ part Cayenne pods.

Dosage Adults: 1 tsp (5ml) 3 times daily (boil off the alcohol), *or* 2 capsules (00 size) 2–3 times daily. Children: over 12 years, adult dose; 9–12 years, ½ adult dose; 1–9 years, ¼ adult dose; younger than 1, ½ tsp (2.5ml) once daily.

Siberian Ginseng is an all-round supportive in the body, and Burdock complements it by stabilizing blood sugar levels, cleansing the bloodstream, neutralizing poisons, and helping the liver, gall bladder, kidneys, and lymph system to work efficiently. Schisandra and Marshmallow boost digestive, nutritional, and energy levels when they are low.

Cayenne helps the other herbs and encourages good circulation.

LEFT *Siberian Ginseng works to support the wellbeing of the whole body.*

43

DIABETES OR HYPOGLYCEMIA

These herbs are predominantly sweet, warming, and slightly bitter, and they strengthen and energize in a sustained and balanced way. This formula, taken in a tincture form, will build stamina over a long period of time, supporting the spleen, pancreas, stomach, and liver.

This formula was created to balance sugar levels, and will support and help those in the early stages of diabetes or who are experiencing hypoglycemia. However, you should consult your doctor or qualified herbalist if you have, or suspect you have, diabetes or hypoglycemia.

ABOVE *Licorice has a sweet root that is widely used in confectionery as well as medicine.*

BELOW *Fenugreek seeds are very popular for medicinal use, especially in India.*

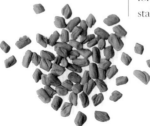

Formula 4 parts Siberian Ginseng root, 4 parts Fenugreek seeds, 2 parts Elecampane seeds, 2 parts Burdock root, 1 part Astragalus root, 1 part Schisandra berries, ½ part Licorice rhizome, ½ part Stevia leaves.

Dosage Adults: 1 tsp (5ml) 3–4 times daily (boil off the alcohol). Children: over 12 years, adult dose; 9–12 years, half adult dose; 1–9 years, quarter adult dose; younger than 1, consult your doctor or qualified herbalist.

Burdock root, Fenugreek seeds, and Elecampane seeds will help to regulate insulin levels.

Fenugreek is one of the oldest of both Western and Eastern plants, and is a favorite in India for the treatment of diabetes. It stabilizes blood sugar levels.

ENERGY SUPPORT

Siberian Ginseng is one of the finest, safest stimulants known in herbal medicine.

Another herb similar in action, but with slight variations, is Pfaffia, sometimes known as Suma and Brazilian Ginseng. In Brazil, Pfaffia is held in high esteem and is used as a cure-all, much like Siberian Ginseng is valued as a panacea. Put Pfaffia and Siberian Ginseng together and you will have a potent combination. If it is difficult to find Pfaffia root, then use Schisandra berries, another very safe, supportive cure-all, from China.

RIGHT *Schisandra berries fight weakness and exhaustion.*

Formula Equal parts of Siberian Ginseng Root and Pfaffia root (or Schisandra berries), *OR* 2 parts Siberian Ginseng root, 1 part Pfaffia Root (or Schisandra berries).

Dosage Adults: 1 tsp (5ml) of tincture 2–4 times daily, depending on the state of energy or whether only general maintenance is required. Children: over 12 years, adult dose; 9–12 years, half adult dose; 1–9 years, quarter adult dose; younger than 1, consult your doctor or a qualified herbalist.

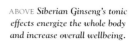

ABOVE *Siberian Ginseng's tonic effects energize the whole body and increase overall wellbeing.*

HEART AND ARTERY REGULATION

This formula combines classic heart and circulatory herbs – Hawthorn, Ginkgo, and Cayenne – with the less traditional and yet superb heart-supportive herbs Siberian Ginseng and Dong Quai.

Formula 3 parts Siberian Ginseng root, 4 parts Hawthorn berries, leaves, and flowers, 2 parts Ginkgo leaves, 1 part Cayenne pods, 1 part Dong Quai root.

Dosage Adults: 1 tsp (5ml) of tincture 3–4 times daily. Children: consult your doctor or other qualified medical practitioner first.

All the herbs in this formula will calm the mind (so often agitated in heart disorders) and will also nourish the blood. Tachycardia, angina, and high blood pressure may be eased with this formula, with safe and positive results. These cases can be as diverse as heightened cholesterol count, blood platelet stickiness which can lead to clumping, and lack of oxygen. However, if you need, or suspect that you may need, heart or artery regulation, you should first consult your doctor or another qualified medical practitioner before taking this formula or any other course of treatment.

CAUTION

If you are pregnant, remove the Dong Quai from these formulas.

NOTE

Other formulas would be needed in order to activate the bowels and relieve any excess water. External application of soothing, warming herbs would also help.

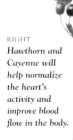

RIGHT
Hawthorn and Cayenne will help normalize the heart's activity and improve blood flow in the body.

RHEUMATISM, ARTHRITIS, ACHING JOINTS AND BONES

These combined herbs, taken as a tincture or in capsule form, will help to motivate circulation, ease inflammation, and provide support for a range of organs and body systems.

Formula 2 parts Siberian Ginseng root, 2 parts Black Cohosh root, 2 parts Devil's Claw root, 2 parts Angelica root, 2 parts Prickly Ash berries or bark, 1 part Cayenne pods, 1 part Dong Quai root.

Dosage Adults: 1 tsp (5ml) 2–4 times daily, or 2 capsules (00 size) 2–3 times daily.

Siberian Ginseng, Black Cohosh, Devil's Claw, Dong Quai, and Angelica help ease the discomfort of the inflammation created by the immune system overworking.

The Prickly Ash and the Cayenne will help circulation. The Siberian Ginseng will support the immune system and help to pace and balance activity while mobility returns so that undue stress is not placed on newly working joints, bones, and tissue.

> **CAUTION**
>
> Avoid this formula if you are pregnant. A qualified herbalist can devise an abridged version for use during pregnancy.

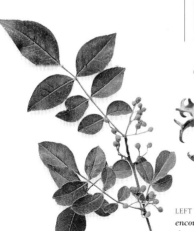

LEFT *Devil's Claw will ease inflammation.*

LEFT *Prickly Ash berries will encourage good circulation and thereby reduce the pain of rheumatism and arthritis.*

Conditions chart

THIS CHART IS *a guide to some of the conditions that Siberian Ginseng can help to treat (see pages 30–36 for dosages) However, this information is not intended to replace medical advice. If you need medical treatment, always consult your doctor or another qualified medical practitioner first.*

NAME	INTERNAL USE
ADRENAL GLAND DISORDERS	Tincture, decoction, tea, capsule
ANXIETY	Tincture, decoction, tea, capsule, wine
APPETITE (LOSS OF)	Tincture, decoction, tea, capsule, wine, soup
ARTHRITIS	Tincture, decoction, tea, capsule, wine
ASTHMA	Tincture, decoctions, tea, capsule
BLOOD PRESSURE PROBLEMS	Tincture, decoction, tea, capsule

NAME	INTERNAL USE
BREASTFEEDING	Tincture, decoction, tea, capsule
CHILDBIRTH	Tincture, decoction, tea, capsule
COUGHS	Tincture, decoction, tea, capsule, soup
CYSTITIS	Tincture, decoction, tea, capsule
DEMENTIA	Tincture, decoction, tea, capsule
DEPRESSION	Tincture, decoction, tea, capsule
DIABETES	Tincture, decoction, tea, capsule, soup
DIGESTION	Tincture, decoction, tea, capsule, soup
ENERGY: BOOST AND MAINTENANCE	Tincture, decoction, tea, capsule
FATIGUE	Tincture, decoction, tea, capsule
FERTILITY	Tincture, decoction, tea, capsule

NAME	INTERNAL USE
HYSTERIA	Tincture, decoction, tea, capsule
IMPOTENCE	Tincture, decoction, tea, capsule
INDIGESTION	Tincture, decoction, tea, capsule, soup, wine
INSOMNIA	Tincture, decoction, tea, capsule
JAUNDICE	Tincture, decoction, tea, capsule
MALNUTRITION	Tincture, decoction, tea, capsule, soup, wine
MENOPAUSE	Tincture, decoction, tea, capsule
MENSTRUATION To "balance"	Tincture, decoction, tea, capsule
MISCARRIAGE To aid recovery afterward	Tincture, decoction, tea, capsule

NAME	INTERNAL USE
NEURALGIA	Tincture, decoction, tea, capsule
NEURASTHENIA	Tincture, decoction, tea, capsule
NEUROSES	Tincture, decoction, tea, capsule
PREGNANCY	Tincture, decoction, tea, capsule, soup
PSORIASIS	Tincture, decoction, tea, capsule
PUBERTY	Tincture, capsule
RHINITIS	Tincture, decoction, tea, capsule
SHINGLES	Tincture, decoction, tea, capsule
SPLEEN DISORDERS	Tincture, decoction, tea, capsule
THYROID PROBLEMS	Tincture, decoction, tea, capsule
TINNITUS	Tincture, decoction, tea, capsule

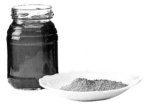

How Siberian Ginseng works

The overall chemistry of Siberian Ginseng produces an effect that is milder and less stimulating than the "regular" Ginsengs such as American and Chinese, but this means the herb is safe for use by a far wider range of people of all ages.

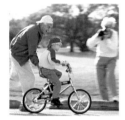

LEFT *Siberian Ginseng is safe for all age groups to take.*

Siberian Ginseng is a true adaptogen — an invigorator of the whole body with no proven unpleasant side effects.

Although Siberian is not a true Ginseng, its action is identical. The genuine Ginsengs contain ginsenocides – which among other effects help nerve regeneration and stimulate various balanced hormonal functions. Like other Ginsengs that are not botanically the same but have many similar actions, Siberian contains many powerful glycosides,

RIGHT *The chemical constituents provide many beneficial effects.*

including eleutherosides and senticosides, which are traceable to its Latin name. It also contains saponins, coumarins, steroids, sterols, triterpenes, a polysaccharide, and lignans. These chemicals have a pharmacological action in the body, which means that the plant will affect all the processes of the body in a unique way.

The glycosides – each of them individual in its behavior – dominate the chemistry of Siberian Ginseng. Among many other functions, they help hormone and immune activity, pain

250
200
150
100

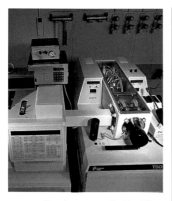

ABOVE *Gas chromatography identifies the chemical composition of plants.*

The steroid constituents of the glycosides provide vital components. They have pain-killing abilities, help endurance, and enhance the ability of the human body to cope with physically difficult situations.

control, inflammation processes, prevent damage by free radicals (see page 55), and aid in the reduction of excess water in the body. Part of their role is to give the adrenal glands extra fuel to work with when in crisis, and then to prevent them from using up any more once the crisis is over. They enforce energy conservation, and the adrenal glands thus manufacture less energy, producing the same amount for better results.

The saponins (and other chemical components) affect the pituitary gland and will therefore balance all the hormonal functions of the human body in both males and females.

RESEARCH RESULTS

In 1964, during clinical testing at the Institute of Biochemistry and Medicine at Khabarovsk, in the former USSR, blood donors were given 4ml of Siberian Ginseng daily. Their hemoglobin levels returned to normal within 13 days, while without the use of Siberian Ginseng this restoration took up to a month.

In 1977, clinical trials of Siberian Ginseng's effect on factory workers were conducted in an area of the Soviet polar region; 1,000 adults were given 4ml of Siberian Ginseng daily for five months. The results, over a year-long period, showed a 40% reduction in days lost from work and a 50% reduction in general sickness.

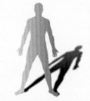

50% REDUCTION IN GENERAL SICKNESS

40% REDUCTION IN WORKING DAYS LOST

PER 1000 POPULATION

ABOVE *Under the Soviet regime, clinical trials proved that Siberian Ginseng improves health and attendance at work.*

MAIN EFFECTS

❋ Stimulates natural cell growth.

❋ Increases red blood cell (and therefore iron) production from bone marrow.

❋ Helps clear blood of alcohol and repairs liver damage from excessive alcohol intake.

❋ Reduces inflammation and enlargement of the prostate gland by altering testosterone levels in the blood.

❋ Increases adrenocorticotrophic hormone production in the pituitary gland, with a knock-on effect to hormones, immune system, and adrenal glands.

CASE STUDY: ALLERGIES

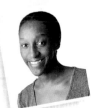

Mary, 35, had a range of allergies that periodically debilitated her. Symptoms ranged from sneezing and a runny nose to raised glands in the neck and "overheating."

After seeing a herbalist, she changed several aspects of her lifestyle, including her diet, and was prescribed a combination of herbs, with Siberian Ginseng as a prominent component. Her allergies gradually abated and became less frequent, and eventually disappeared altogether.

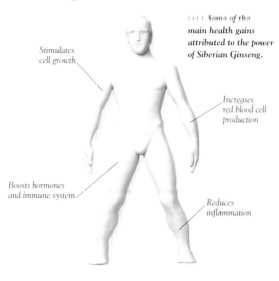

LEFT *Some of the* **main health gains attributed to the power of Siberian Ginseng.**

Stimulates cell growth

Increases red blood cell production

Boosts hormones and immune system

Reduces inflammation

Glossary

ADAPTOGENIC

Herb that empowers the whole body in a non-specific way, and with no unpleasant side effects.

AMPHOTERIC

In herbal terms, a herb that knows where to go in the body, and for what purpose.

ANTIOXIDANTS

Understood in current models of immunity, these substances (found particularly in high-chlorophyll foods) protect the cells from damaging free radicals, which themselves have been created through oxygenation. In simple terms, it is rather like preventing metal from rusting.

ARTERIOSCLEROSIS

Hardening of the arteries.

BURLAP

Universally used type of herb storage bag that allows the contents to breathe.

CHOLESTEROL

A fatlike substance in the blood and most tissues, especially nervous tissue. Cholesterol is synthesized in the body from acetate, mainly in the liver.

CORTISONE

Drug that mimics the action of corticosteroids – any of several hormones found in the cortex of the adrenal glands.

COUMARINS

Blood thinning agents.

ESTROGEN

Female reproductive system hormone; production in the body is lessened during the menopause.

EXTRASYSTOLE

Common irregularity of the heart (dropped beat).

FREE RADICALS

Highly reactive particles that damage cell membranes, DNA, and other cellular structures.

GERMINATION

When the seed has produced a primordial root below and has emerging leaves.

HOMEOSTASIS

Process of maintaining constant physical and emotional conditions despite external changes – the primary function of most organs in the body.

HUMUS
See leaf mold.

HYPERTONICITY
Maintaining vascular system tone and elasticity.

HYPOGLYCEMIA
Low blood sugar, causing muscle weakness, confusion, and sweating.

IMMUNITY
Capacity and function of the body to fend off foreign bodies (fungi, viruses, bacteria), and/or disarm and eject them.

LACTATION
Breastfeeding.

LEAF MOLD
Leaves that are collected in the fall and allowed to decay in order to provide nutrition and bulk to growing plants in pots or flower-beds; sometimes referred to as "leaf litter."

LEUCOCYTOSIS
Increase in the number of white blood cells in the blood (leucocytes), a characteristic of many infections and disorders, including leukemia

LIGNANS
Woody parts of the plant.

LYMPHOCYTE
Type of white blood cell.

METASTASIS
Migration of disease, such as with bacterial infection or cancer.

NEONATAL
Concerning newborn babies, conventionally limited to the first four weeks of life.

NEURALGIA
Pain originating in any nerve.

NEURASTHENIA
Inflammation of a nerve.

NEUROTRANSMITTERS
Molecules released into the synaptic cleft in response to nerve impulse.

PANCREATITIS
Inflammation of the pancreas.

PATHOGEN
Microbe capable of causing disease.

PHOTOSYNTHESIS
Process by which green plants utilize energy from the sun to produce food from carbon dioxide and water.

PHYSIOLOGICAL
Functions and phenomena of living organs and their individual parts.

PLATELETS

Disk-shaped fragments enclosed in cell membranes that flow through the blood and promote clotting.

POLYSACCHARIDES

Group of sugars.

PSYCHOSIS

One of a group of mental disorders involving loss of touch with reality.

RHINITIS

Inflammation of the lining of the nose.

RHIZOME

Underground stem (root) that grows horizontally.

RNA SYNTHESIS

Process of making ribonucleic acid.

SAPONIN

Chemical plant component, characteristically producing a foam, that is a frequent part of plant hormone activity.

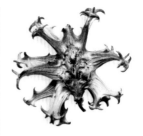

SCHIZOPHRENIA

Type of psychosis or mental derangement that is characterized by delusions and hallucinations, as well as a disintegration of the process of thinking, of contact with reality, and of emotional responsiveness.

SENTICOSIDE

Chemical component responsible for hormonal activity in both the plant and the human body.

STEROIDS

In the case of Siberian Ginseng, plant chemicals similar to those that are formed naturally in the adrenal glands.

TACHYCARDIA

Unduly rapid heartbeat.

TRIGLYCERIDES

Three chain carboxylic or fatty acids that are important energy storage molecules. Triglycerides are formed from digested dietary fat and are the form in which fat is stored in the body.

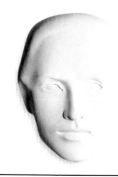

Further reading

AMERICAN GINSENG: A GROWERS GUIDE, HISTORY AND USE, W. Scott Persons (Bright Mountain Books, 1994)

BRITISH HERBAL PHARMACOPOEIA 1996 (British Herbal Medical Association, 1996)

CHEMISTRY OF LIFE, Steven Rose (Georgetown Press, 1984)

CHINESE MEDICINAL HERBS, Li Shih Chen (Georgetown Press, 1973)

COMPLETE ILLUSTRATED HOLISTIC HERBAL, D. Hoffmann (Element Books, 1996)

ELEUTHEROCOCCUS SENTICOSUS, Bruce Halstead & Loretta Hood (Oriental Healing Arts Institute, 1984

ENCYCLOPAEDIA OF HERBS AND HERBALISM, Malcolm Stuart (Black Cat, 1987)

ENCYCLOPAEDIA OF HERBS AND THEIR USES, Deni Bown (Dorling Kindersley, 1995)

ENCYCLOPEDIA OF MEDICINAL PLANTS, Andrew Chevallier (Dorling Kindersley, 1996)

ESSENTIAL SCIENCE CHEMISTRY, Freemantle & Tidy (Oxford University Press, 1983)

FOUNDATIONS OF HEALTH, Christopher Hobbs (Botanica Press, 1992)

GARDENER'S DICTIONARY OF PLANT NAMES, A.W. Smith (Cassell, 1971)

GINSENG, Christopher Hobbs (Botanica Press, 1996)

HERBAL PHARMACOLOGY, Christopher Hobbs (Botanica Press, 1996)

HERBS OF LIFE, Lesley Tierra (The Crossing Press, 1992)

ILLUSTRATED ENCYCLOPAEDIA OF HERBS, (Chandler Press, 1984)

MANUAL OF CONVENTIONAL MEDICINE FOR ALTERNATIVE PRACTITIONERS, Stephen Gascoigne (Jigame Press, 1994)

MEDICAL ENCYCLOPAEDIA, Peter Wingate (Penguin, 1972)

NUTRITIONAL HERBOLOGY, Mark Pederson (Wendell W. Whitman Company, 1994)

OUT OF THIS EARTH, Simon Mills (Viking, 1991)

PLANETARY HERBOLOGY, Michael Tierra (Lotus Press, 1988)

PLANT PHYSIOLOGY IN RELATION TO HORTICULTURE, J. K. A. Bleaside (Macmillan, 1973)

PRINCIPLES OF ANATOMY AND PHYSIOLOGY, Tortora, Reynolds & Grabowski (HarperCollins, 1996)

SCHOOL OF NATURAL HEALING, Dr. Christopher (Christopher Publications, 1976)

SOILS AND OTHER GROWTH MEDIA, A.W. Flegman (Macmillan, 1975)

SPIRITUAL PROPERTIES OF HERBS, Gurudas (Cassandra Press, 1988)

TEXTBOOK OF ADVANCED HERBOLOGY, Terry Willard (Wild Rose College of Natural Healing, 1992)

TEXTBOOK OF MODERN HERBOLOGY, Terry Willard (Wild Rose College of Natural Healing, 1993)

Useful addresses

**British Herbal Medicine
Association (B.H.M.A)**
Sun House, Church Street, Stroud,
Glos. GL5 1JL, UK
Tel: 011 44 1453–751389
Fax: 011 44 1453–751402
Works with the Medicine Control
Agency to promote high standards of
quality and safety of herbal medicine

Herb Society
Deddington Hill Farm,
Warmington, Banbury,
Oxon OX17 1XB, UK
Tel: 011 44 1295–692000
Fax: 011 44 1295–692004
Educational charity that disseminates
information about herbs and
organizes workshops

**The Wild Plant Conservation
Charity**
The Natural History Museum
Cromwell Road,
London SW7 5BD, UK
Tel: 011 44 171–938 9123
Registered charity to save British
wild plants

SUPPLIERS IN THE UK

Baldwin & Company
171–173 Walworth Road,
London SE17 1RW, UK
Tel: 011 44 171–703 5550
Herbs, storage bottles, jars, and
containers available

Hambleden Herbs
Court Farm, Milverton,
Somerset TA4 1NF, UK
Tel: 011 44 1823–401205
Organic herbs by mail order

Herbs, Hands, Healing
The Cabins, Station Warehouse,
Station Road, Pulham Market,
Norfolk IP21 4XF, UK
Tel: 011 44 1379–608007
Tel/fax: 011 44 1379–608201
Herbal formulas, organic herbs,
and Superfood

SUPPLIERS/SCHOOLS IN THE USA

American Botanical Pharmacy
PO Box 3027, Santa Monica,
CA 90408, USA
Tel/fax: 1310 453–1987
Manufacturer and distributor of
herbal products; runs training courses

Blessed Herbs
109 Barre Plains Road,
Oakham,
MA 01068, USA
Tel: 1800-489–4372
Dried bulk herbs are available by
mail order in order to make your
own preparations

United Plant Savers
PO Box 420,
East Barre,
VT 05649, USA
Aims to preserve wild Native
American medicinal plants

Other Healing Herb Books
in the Nutshell Series

❧

ECHINACEA
ECHINACEA ANGUSTIFOLIA
ECHINACEA PURPUREA

❧

GARLIC
ALLIUM SATIVUM

❧

GINKGO
GINKGO BILOBA

❧

HAWTHORN
CRATAEGUS MONOGYNA

❧

MARIGOLD
CALENDULA OFFICINALIS

❧

ST. JOHN'S WORT
HYPERICUM PERFORATUM

❧

SAW PALMETTO
SERENOA SERRULATA

❧